COPYRIGHT

I0490322

Table of Contents

A MESSAGE TO YOU!

In early 1994, Sandra met a beautiful 27-year-old woman. She was perfect in every way. Friendly, happy, and warm. Under the surface, however, lived a fragile young girl scared to come to the light. Her reflections came out in the form of dry, flushed hands. The otherwise, confident young 27-year-old damsel felt the daunting urge to wash off the contact of everything. Her soul was crippled with shackles forcing her to hide away and not talk about it. She always appeared happy and positive around others. She almost had it all together, almost.

Deep inside, she was tormented, haunted by the voices in her head feeding her fears of contracting a deadly sickness and making others sick. Those thoughts and images in her head dominated her mind until she refused to stay at home and hide away, any longer. She refused to fuel any more power to OCD. Realizing the only way out of fear is through it, was the moment everything changed.

This damsel in distress wasn't looking for a prince, she was looking for a sword. She was looking to be her very own hero. She decided to face her fears – to make herself uncomfortable. She decided to not give in to her tears and pain, refusing her desire to go back hiding in her perfectly sanitized bedroom.

Years later, she became a beacon of hope for hundreds of people suffering from OCD, anxiety, and depression. This is the story of Sandra – our founder and visionary. At Sandra Wallace Inc., we help people live their lives with the pulsating energy and the vigour they truly deserve.

FOREWORD

It's a problem for me that so many people are living a life of quiet desperation as a result of the impact that Obsessive Compulsive Disorder (OCD) has had on their life. I solve that problem because it used to be me. It was the worst time of my life. With God's grace, having OCD allows me to go and serve others. What is clear to me now, is that I have a mission along with a purpose to help those who continue to suffer as I once did.

WHAT OTHERS ARE SAYING ABOUT SANDRA AND HER COACHING STRATEGIES

"I am a clinical psychologist specializing in Obsessive Compulsive Disorder (OCD). On September 15, 1994, I began providing Cognitive Behaviour Therapy (CBT) focusing on prolonged exposure to Sandra Wallace. Sandra's OCD was severe. She had a wide range of fears of contamination, accidentally hurting strangers, writing inappropriate comments on documents, and to authority figures such as the police to name a few. Initially, I provided treatment once or twice a week often accompanying her to her various feared locations. She worked diligently and consistently to overcome her fears by complying with homework tasks that we agreed on at the end of each session. She would then tackle the agreed-upon assignments on her own between treatment sessions and kept detailed records of her progress. In my 30 years of providing CBT to clients with OCD, I can honestly say that I have never witnessed anyone work so hard at overcoming her fears. She tackled each one systematically and with grace. As the years went by, I saw her blossom into the person she wanted to be. That is, helping others who had OCD by volunteering her time with the OCD Foundation of MB and eventually starting a business treating others with OCD. Sandra knows as much about the pain of experiencing symptoms of OCD and treatment with CBT as many professionals who specialize in this debilitating disorder. I commend her on her work and have no hesitation in recommending her to others."

- Dr. Vivienne C. Rowan, Ph.D. | Clinical Psychologist

"As an inpatient psychiatrist, I have had the privilege of working with Ms. Wallace in a variety of clinical settings including acute care and psychiatric rehabilitation. She has demonstrated a dedication to prioritizing the patient's needs and applying her professional knowledge and skills. Her gentle temperament is an attribute that does not go unnoticed. Her clinical teaching skills with students are highly respected. It is a pleasure to continue working with her."

- Dr. Roger Graham M.D. | *FRCPC Psychiatry*

"Sandra's program has changed my life and for the first time has made me challenge my OCD instead of living victim to it. Her insight into changing the way your brain functions is key to understanding how to beat your OCD. Her 5-week program puts you in a rhythm that then carries over into your everyday life, making it possible to overcome your thoughts and allow you to live a life that is not shackled down by obtrusive thoughts. I am now medication free after 5 years thanks to Sandra and her dedication to helping people with OCD."

- Melissa | *Program Successor*

"Sandra Wallace has made a huge impact on my life. I have struggled with OCD for about 15 years and have dealt with different subtypes and triggers related to my OCD. Doing the 5-week express recovery program with Sandra made the greatest impact on my mental health. I went from feeling debilitated and controlled by OCD, to having confidence in myself and making real day-to-day changes. The fears that I have overcome with Sandra have changed my life and I finally feel like I am supported and making positive changes. Sandra was someone with whom I felt supported and respected, and I always knew I could tell her anything free of judgment. Sandra has become someone I trust and the treatment she provides plays a pivotal role in my recovery. With Sandra by my side and the tools I have been able to take away from the program, I now feel like I can take on whatever OCD throws at me. Fighting OCD doesn't come naturally, I had to continuously work hard to make it happen. Sandra gave me the tools to be able to do that, and I have never felt so brave."

- Hunter Pickering | Program Successor

"My experience working with Sandra as a coach has been exceptional. I have seen a few different counsellors and psychologists over the years, but the coaching, support, and tools I received from Sandra to work through my anxiety have been far more practical and helpful than typical "therapy". I recommend her to anyone struggling with any type of anxiety."

- Allison | Program Successor

"I really enjoyed working with Sandra. She was very thorough right from the beginning and took the time to understand all of the OCD challenges I was dealing with. Most importantly, she gave me tangible things to work on every week and I saw real progress. I felt entirely comfortable describing my behaviour to her because I knew she had gone through her own challenges. My OCD has improved thanks to my sessions with Sandra and I look forward to staying in touch and seeking her guidance in the future.

Nolan | Program Successor

"I have known Sandra for roughly 10 years and knew from the minute I met her; she would be in my life. I recall our first meeting and how attentive she was to me, not allowing anything external to sway her from our conversation. This trait of Sandra's personality was not a one-time refection, it is a part of who she is as a person. Her passion to connect with people and help them in any way she can is as genuine as her scintillating smile. Her family and friends are such an integral part of her life with her always exploring ways to connect with each and every one of them.

Sandra, as a friend, is the epitome of friendship. She's non-judgmental, open- minded, genuine, compassionate, and level-headed. She can always be counted on to listen and offer support when needed. Her wonderful sense of humour, drive for adventure, and personal life experiences have gifted her the ability to see any situation with a lens of fierce optimism. I believe people come into our lives for a reason, a season, or a lifetime and Sandra is a lifetime friend.

Sandra's strength lies in her passion to help one and all and her desire to follow ethical guidelines to ensure trust, and professionalism when building rapport with clients. As a client and a friend, I appreciated her gentle, grounded process which provided me with peace of mind, clarity, and a new perspective on an issue that was troubling me. I was left with a feeling of energy and new founded meaning and purpose."

-JP | MA RPC

"I have had the pleasure of subcontracting Sandra to do lectures for my college in the Community Support Worker Program. Sandra was both diligent and knowledgeable about the material and was invaluable in assisting my students to take the next step in education and information to the 'next level'. She has also taught me many valuable tips for working both professionally, and personally, and trust she can do the same for you. I look forward to working with Sandra again and I highly encourage anyone to use Sandra's services in any facet (learning, teaching, or counselling) as I am confident, she can do the same for you and/or your organization."

- Lloyd Richard | College Instructor

"Listening to Sandra's story has been one of the most inspirational experiences of my life. She has fought through the most trying times of her OCD experience and come out as a shining beacon of hope for millions of people waiting for their breakthrough moment. Through her journey, she has documented a myriad of wins and setbacks that propelled her transformation. Despite all the incredible work she has done in the field to help her patients and clients, Sandra remains curious to learn, question, and explore more. I have seen Sandra researching for hours to help her clients with the most complex challenges. She gets invested in the lives and healing journey of her clients. Her remarkable work ethic and her selfless commitment to the field of Mental health are what make Sandra a Coach."

- Noor Pannu | Digital Marketing Strategist

"I am privileged to have known Sandra for the last 7 yrs. It is very obvious, whether speaking in person or via phone, that Sandra's passion for mental health shines through with every word. Sandra continues to make a difference with not just every course she delivers as a Mental Health First Aid instructor but with every interaction, she has with others. Sandra through her passion, knowledge, and experience truly enriches the lives of those around her."

- Denise Waligora B.S., | *Training & Delivery Specialist* | *Mental Health First Aid, Canada*

"As an academic in the healthcare industry and a lover of learning myself, I have had the opportunity to attend various lectures where Sandra has been the instructor or keynote presenter and I can tell you - she is a rare find - a leader in the area of OCD who not only demonstrates passion and commitment for learning herself but with a laser focus to vehemently convey that information into the minds of others. She is an invaluable resource to those who suffer in the world of Obsessions and Compulsions with a unique ability to provide candour and compassion to those in need."

- HJ | *Pharmacist*

"I recently had the opportunity to attend a course taught by Sandra. Sandra came well prepared for the task at hand. She engaged all the participants keeping the day lively and interesting. Her knowledge and enthusiasm encouraged me to learn more. Time spent with Sandra was time well spent."

- Collette Moss | *Pharmacy Technician*

"I have completed the 10 weeks of OCD therapy program with Sandra Wallace. I found that the trigger analysis should start sooner at the beginning of the few weeks instead of toward the end. The program should extend to 15 weeks instead of 10 weeks. Sandra is a good listener and the advice I learned from her was useful."

- Anonymous | *Program Successor*

"Sandra is wonderful, as a person and professional. She loves to see others succeed in life. Right off the bat, you can tell she is caring and friendly - Her smile is infectious and she makes it really easy to open up to her. She has helped me in more ways than she knows; and for that, Sandra is not only my co-worker but also my friend."

- Cecilia Bautista | *Registered Psych Nurse*

"I have been teaching along with Sandra for over 6 years. She's not only an amazing teacher but an amazing mentor to her co-facilitators. Sandra speaks from the heart and isn't afraid of using personal experiences to ramp up the learning experience for her students. Sandra is very professional, yet personable. She understands the importance of adult earning and how it requires a lot of flexibility and preparation. She can go with the flow and change up her curriculum when need be. I always look forward to when I get to teach with Sandra."

- Lacey | *Healthcare Professional*

"Sandra's way of teaching and delivering the message is really attractive. She uses all possible tools to do it - videos, leaflets, and references. The classroom is not just another boring 8 hours of listening. She gets everybody in the class to share in - playing games that facilitate understanding and an enriched learning experience. With Sandra, you forget to look at your watch waiting for the class hours to pass. The time glides away smoothly before you can notice. Sandra's voice modulations eliminate any chance of monotony while drawing attention. She is just so very positive, always smiling, brings pulsating energy to each class leaving her audience enthralled."

- Mina | *Pharmacy M*

Motivate And Inspire Others!

Share This Book

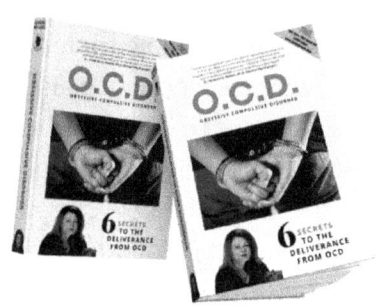

Special Quantities:

5-20 Books	$21.95 USD
21-99 Books	$18.95 USD
100-499 Books	$15.95 USD
500-999 Books	$10.95 USD
1000+ Books	$8.95 USD

Retail Price: $24.95 USD

TO PLACE AN ORDER:
Cell/Text- 1-204-295-4408
Email- info@theocdcoach.com
Website- www.TheOCDCoach.com

The Ideal Professional Speaker for Your Next Event!

Any organization that wants to develop their people to become extraordinary, needs to hire Sandra for a keynote and/or workshop training!

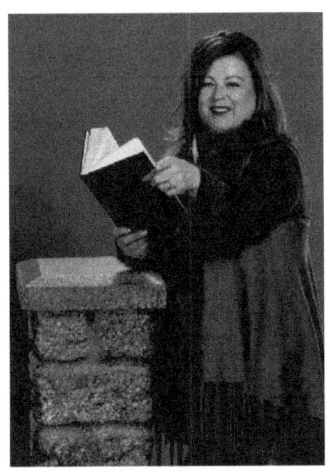

TO CONTACT OR BOOK SANDRA TO SPEAK:

Sandra Wallace Inc.
PO Box 10021 RPO South Selkirk, Manitoba R1A 0P5 Canada
Cell/Text- 1-204-295-4408
Email- info@theocdcoach.com
Website- www.TheOCDCoach.com

The Ideal Coach for You!

If you're ready to overcome challenges, have major breakthroughs, and achieve higher levels, then you will love having Sandra as your Coach!

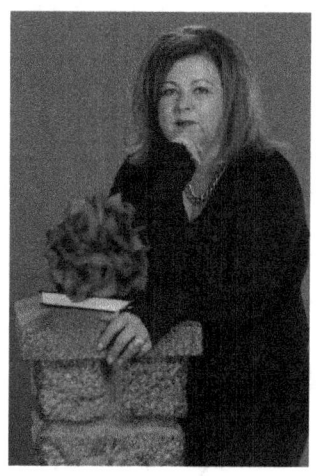

TO CONTACT OR BOOK SANDRA TO COACH:

Sandra Wallace Inc.
PO Box 10021
RPO South
Selkirk, Manitoba
R1A 0P5 Canada
Cell/Text- 1-204-295-4408
Email- info@theocdcoach.com
Website- www.TheOCDCoach.com

DEDICATIONS

It is with respect, admiration, and sincere appreciation, that I dedicate this book to my wonderful family. Without you and the lessons you have taught me throughout my life, I would not have the blessing of being where I am today. Thank you from the bottom of my heart! I love you dearly!

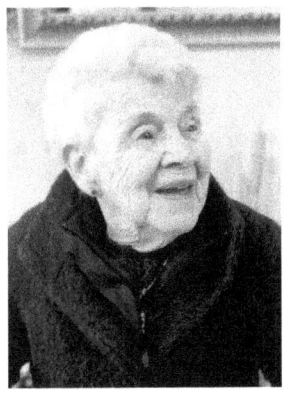

Doreen Mary Pomozybida

This book was created during the time I was caring for my precious mamma. Many times, spent lying next to her while she napped or at the edge of her bed recording my words and ideas for this book. My father loved me in his own way but my mamma loved me in many ways. Mamma was the one who taught me to respect others. Whenever she saw someone hurt or in need of help, she would say "That's someone's daughter or someone's son". She always encouraged us to love one another unconditionally. She is one of my greatest motivators to go out to the world and reach those living a silent life of desperation.

Mamma, you are my angel, I thank you for looking over me, always! 🖤

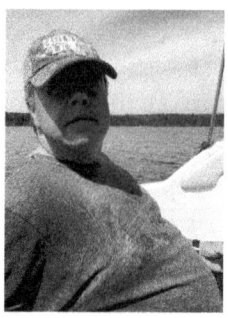

Randy Bernard Pomozybida

I want to acknowledge and thank my brother for all the support he provided me through the years of living with OCD. There were times when I was very debilitated from OCD and could not drive, go alone to a store, or carry on my daily activities. Randy would do whatever he could to help me in these times. Although, it was difficult for him to understand why I did the things I did, he loved me just the same. OCD is so embarrassing, shameful, and guilt-ridden, it was hard for me to let others in and see my compulsions.

Thank you, Randy, for loving me unconditionally. I love you! 🖤

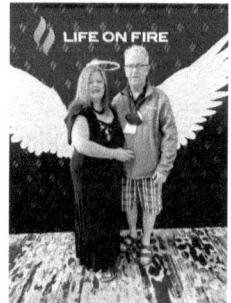

To my husband who has stood by me unconditionally and waited patiently for me as I did my compulsions, "Just one more time?" My OCD was at its worst during our first several years of marriage, he has continued to support me with love, kindness, and understanding, even in times it may be difficult to comprehend. He has been my steadfast rock since the beginning. Together we will keep OCD at bay till the end of time! Love you! ♥

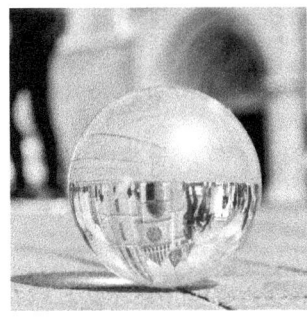

To my clients and those of you, I have yet to meet

For those whom I have had the privilege and opportunity to work with as your coach, thank you!! I have truly learned so much from each person I have worked with. Much of the learning came in the way of pain, torment, confusion, shame, and guilt. It was your willingness to be vulnerable, that allowed us to push through this thing called OCD. It is because of you, yes you reading this, that I have dedicated the rest of my life to helping others living with OCD to rise above the obsessions and resist the compulsions.

"I will meet you there!"

Acknowledgements

This book has been made possible only because of the decades of studying OCD and attending the International Obsessive-Compulsive Foundation (IOCDF) Annual Conference for 14 years. The opportunity to learn from the best of the best, the pioneers of OCD that shared their expertise on how to overcome OCD step-by-step. I am especially grateful to Dr. Jonathan Grayson PhD, Dr. Edna Foa PhD, Dr. Fred Penzel PhD, Dr. Bruce Hyman PhD, and Cherry Pedrick R.N. for their years of dedication to the advancement of the awareness and treatment of OCD. Through various platforms I have had ample opportunities to spend time with these experts in the realm of OCD. As a result, I was able to learn, implement and apply techniques successfully in my own life. This led me to help coach others through a variety of programs I created.

I also want to express a heartfelt thank you to Dr. Vivian Rowan PhD, Psych. for all the many years of support and guidance in my journey with Cognitive Behaviour Therapy (CBT) and Exposure Response Prevention (ERP).

My greatest gratitude comes from the lessons taught to me by the many patients I have had the pleasure of working with over the years. As a Registered Psychiatric Nurse RPN for the last 28 years, as well as my personal 1:1 clients whom I have coached, it is because of YOU I have learned to be courageous, thankful, and always grateful for each day.

To some of my greatest mentors, thank you for your willingness to be vulnerable and persistent in teaching me how to do the same. Les Brown, Tony Robbins, Dean Graziosi, Brené Brown, Lisa Nichols, Dr. Sonya Stribling, Jeanine Blackwell, Nick and Megan Unsworth and James Malinchak.

Noor Pannu

I want to say for the last several years one of my greatest motivators has been you, Noor. We met out of fate and our working relationship started with a dream to build my business to help others on a journey of OCD. Noor, you helped me to see the strengths in me that I never knew I had. There have been endless hours devoted to my mission through your hard work and expertise. Thank you, Noor, for believing in me and wanting this just as much as I did!!!

Mathieu Castel

To my dear friend Mat who is practically on the other side of the world literally from me, I want to thank you.! You have been an inspiration for me in wanting to write my book by facilitating all of the behind-the-scenes work that you make seem so easy! Thank you for all the direction and guidance you have given me in making some very big decisions in my business operations. It continues to be a privilege to work with you. I can't wait for our next adventure and creation!

Evelyn Visperas

Evelyn, we have done so much in such a short time of working together. Having you join our team has been one of the best highlights since the onset of our journey at The OCD Coach. You have talents and gifts that touch all aspects of the operation, and that go beyond what I could have wished for. Thank you for being willing to take on new initiatives especially for helping me step by step with this book. I cannot wait to see all the magic as we do more amazing work together!

Jo-Ann Wolloff

Jo-Ann you have been a part of my Life on Fire Family since I joined just over a year ago. The opportunity to spend 1:1 time with you as you gently guide me in decision-making and goal-setting makes me want to hold myself accountable to not only myself but to others. I have learned to lead by example and do things even when I'm scared. Thank you for your knowledge and insight into the world of technology. Together, we are stewards in Christ.

CHAPTER 1 OUTLINE

HOW DO YOU KNOW YOU HAVE THIS THING CALLED OCD?

- What are obsessions & compulsions?

- How do you alleviate the anxiety?

- The clock will always STRIKE 12.

- How to jump out of the vicious cycle?

- It is important to get an official diagnosis by an appropriate professional.

- Assessment Tools to help dive further into my signs and symptoms.

CHAPTER 1
HOW DO YOU KNOW YOU HAVE THIS THING CALLED OCD?

No one knows exactly what causes OCD. The obsessions are thoughts, urges and impulses that are unwanted and often very intrusive. The obsessions provoke high anxiety and distress, you feel compelled to perform a compulsion/ritual to alleviate the anxiety and neutralize the fears driven by the obsession. The number one motivation in this process is a person's fear of the possible consequences. YOU desire 100% certainty that the feared obsession will not come to fruition.

Unfortunately, none of us can ever be guaranteed 100% certainty of anything in life. This is, without doubt, the number one challenge in helping the person living with OCD to understand this concept. The only way to overcome OCD is living with uncertainty, and in many cases the low probability that the feared situation will occur - but again, this is not a zero probability. That, right there, is hard for a person living with OCD to accept. When I am speaking to audiences about how OCD encourages and insists that you be 100% certain, it is then you must be reminded to take the risk that OCD says you should not take. By doing so you create opportunities for uncertainty.

A great deal of time is spent on obsessions and performing the compulsions. A minimum of one hour a day but often much more time is consumed daily. When I am doing my intakes 1:1 with clients, they often reveal the amount of time spent doing compulsions which can be very time consuming, often occupying 6-8 hours daily.

OCD can result from a combination of genetically inherited tendencies or predispositions combined with significant environmental factors. The onset of OCD symptoms is usually gradual, although some people have reported sudden onsets. It is not uncommon for symptoms of OCD to go up during times of emotional stress. The obsessions can bring on plenty of stress and significant impairment in functioning.

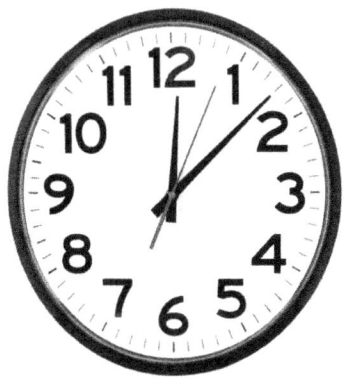

The Clock will ALWAYS strike 12 again!

The clock strikes 12 and you have an obsession which often comes in the form of a disturbing trigger.

At 12:15 this produces emotions causing tremendous anxiety.

At 12:30 there is this overwhelming need to perform a compulsion/ritual which is intended to alleviate your anxiety.

At 12:45, you have some sense of relief and your anxiety lessens. It is very important to remember that the relief is only TEMPORARY.

It is only a matter of when, not if, the next obsession rears its ugly face. The clock will strike 12 again and this whole vicious cycle will start over.

You need to learn to jump out of the cycle seeing things from an objective point of view at 12:08.

The following are some examples of exploring your symptoms further to gain more insight into OCD:

- Yale – Brown Obsessive Compulsive Scale - developed by Wayne Goodman, Psychiatrist.
- Y-BOCS symptom checklist.
- Obsessive Concerns Checklist - Freedom From Obsessive Compulsive Disorder: A Personalized Recovery Program for Living with Uncertainty by Jonathan Grayson PhD. Berkely/Penguin Press. NY. 2014. Adapted and Modified from Obsessive Compulsive Disorders: A Complete Guide to Getting Well And Staying Well by Fred Penzel PhD.
- Compulsive Activities Checklist - Freedom From Obsessive Compulsive Disorder: A Personalized Recovery Program for Living with Uncertainty by Jonathan Grayson PhD. Berkely/Penguin Press. NY. 2014. Adapted and Modified from Obsessive Compulsive Disorders: A Complete Guide to Getting Well And Staying Well by Fred Penzel PhD.
- Obsessional Beliefs Questionnaire.
- Self OCD List.

**It is essential to have a professional assess and officially diagnosis you as having OCD.

CHAPTER 2 OUTLINE

THE GOLD STANDARD TREATMENT COGNITIVE THERAPY (CBT)

- Cognitive Behaviour Therapy (CBT).

- Exposure Response Prevention (ERP).

- Types of Exposures.

- Know your Triggers.

CHAPTER 2
THE GOLD STANDARD TREATMENT
COGNITIVE THERAPY (CBT)

Cognitive Behaviour Therapy (CBT)

Cognitive Behaviour Therapy was initiated in the 1970's and rose to become the Gold Standard Treatment for OCD. Today it is still the number one treatment modality in overcoming OCD. Within CBT lies the number one Technique referred to as Exposure Response Prevention (ERP). This stand-alone technique involves gradual exposure to feared situations or thoughts. Slowly and consistently, you break down the walls of what can be an incredibly debilitating disorder.

CBT refers to specific methods and techniques that help change your faulty ideas and beliefs. In essence, if you can change the way you perceive your reality around you, it will ultimately change your behaviour.

Exposure Response Prevention (ERP)

Let's break down this acronym ERP. What does the E stand for? It stands for Exposure to the much-feared situation, place or object that triggers your OCD. Response Prevention, on the other hand, is exactly what it says; you want to prevent yourself from responding by doing a compulsion to alleviate the anxiety that is brought on by the obsession. You deliberately want to put yourselves in a situation without performing a compulsion. Wow! Isn't that scary? But overtime you will come to realize that the very thing you feared will not necessarily occur if you don't do the compulsion.

Somebody once explained it to me this way, your thoughts are like a bus, you can watch the thoughts come and get on and ride them, or you can allow them to come and go. If you do choose to get on the bus, you can ring and get off at any time. You can actually allow your thoughts to come and go reinforcing that there is no obligation to the thoughts, they are simply thoughts. This is really hard sometimes, depending on the situation that you are presently in. Please be courageous, take that risk, and trust that over time, it's going to get easier.

Studies show over several years, approximately 75% of individuals who went through an intense treatment program achieved substantial relief and more importantly retained their gains for at least 18 months following treatment.

What are the types of exposure?

There are two basic types of exposures:

IN VIVO - refers to the direct confrontation of activities, feared objects or situations. Situations where this type of exposure may be used is in-person and real-life events. It is important to work with a trained professional to develop a hierarchy of your obsessions and compulsions.

IMAGINAL - refers to exposure of your fears and fearful situations by recording in your own voice a script with a detailed description of the event/outcome as it relates to your obsession. This will allow it to be brought to life as the story unfolds. In this way you are confronting the feared thought and consequences using your imagination.

Ideally, it would be nice if you could do it all in vivo, but there are certain circumstances where that is not applicable. In my case, I'll use my example of the "Hit and Run OCD". Obviously, I was not able to go out and practice by hitting individuals on the road or sidewalk, I had to create other ways to follow through with my ERP when it came to that type of OCD. Each script ends in catastrophic outcomes. Another way to look at imaginal exposure is by looking at it like scripting. This involves confronting the feared thought and consequences using your imagination. It really must be done in a certain format in order to be effective.

What I mean by that is it must invoke some kind of distress as an actual obsession would. In this type of exposure, be mindful, it is crucial to have fear eliciting triggers, as you're doing the imaginal script.

Know your triggers-Be mindful of your triggers as they are very important.

Let's cover some of the ways that you can identify your triggers. The triggers can occur in a variety of situations. Stress can bring on triggers and increase their intensity. These can involve a variety of situations, depending on what type of OCD you have. What you're exposed to on a daily basis may also influence the number of triggers. Sometimes they come to you more frequently when feeling tired or later in the day. I notice if I have a lot on my mind or I'm going through a stressful time in my life, OCD comes out to play full out and often with greater intensity.

Depending where you're at in your ERP, and your comfort level, when you have a trigger, you may use that as an opportunity to expose yourself to the trigger and practice ERP. I find myself doing that still to this day. If a thought comes to mind and I'm looking at possibly doing a ritual, then I will purposely set myself up to be exposed to the very thing that is causing my anxiety and refrain from doing the compulsion.

CHAPTER 3 OUTLINE
IMPORTANCE OF WORKING WITH A COACH

- Importance of working with an expert Coach in OCD.

- Readiness.

- Roadmap.

- Courage.

CHAPTER 3
IMPORTANCE OF WORKING WITH A COACH

A good coach must be trained in CBT, more specifically Cognitive Behavioural methods, and ERP. The more one learns about CBT and ERP, the more beneficial it can be in determining if the current modalities are effective. With time, you should see your anxiety decrease as well as be able to refrain from performing rituals whether they are mental rituals or otherwise. A coach who has expertise in OCD, will be well-educated and have knowledge of the specific questions to ask to help gain a greater understanding of your specific types of OCD. This is key in order to provide the best possible outcomes and treatment plan to set you up for success. Your coach should be able to understand OCD and the benefit of the treatment but more importantly, know at what pace to integrate the techniques and to course- correct if the desired results are not yet obtained. All of these are factors and are a must.

Creating and designing a tailor-made program very specific to your needs is where my expertise lies as your coach. When I am working with my clients 1:1 we are able to create a very specific program that they are comfortable agreeing to and create a gradual hierarchy to allow for CBT and ERP to take place. Having the background that I have for the past 28 years, both from a personal and professional level, I can help simplify the requirements to allow for course correction during your ERP, should we find that what you're doing is not producing satisfactory outcomes.

Having gone through the ERP first hand with a 99.9% success rate 28 years ago, following and completing an intensive course of therapy, this has allowed me to realize what the things were that were prohibiting me from reaching my goals and desires. This experience may provide you with the same clues.

As your coach, I am able to see your obsessions, triggers, anxiety, and fears from a more objective perspective. I am also able to help you to determine what the compulsions are as they relate to each of your obsessions.

It is important to emphasize the fact that you do not have to accept the apparent meaning of your thoughts - just the fact that you have them. The only real meaning behind your thoughts is that they have created a tremendous amount of anxiety. When working 1:1 with my clients, we deal with the emotions brought on by the thoughts and learn to work through the emotional piece, while shifting the mindset.

Readiness

The very first thing is you must be mindful of your readiness, insight, and your motivation. Let's go back to the very beginning when we discussed the vicious cycle of OCD, and the importance of jumping out of that cycle prior to responding to your obsessions. Your approach, now going forward, must be very different. You need to recognize that suppressing the thoughts and/or doing a compulsion will only make the thoughts worse over time. I can't emphasize that enough, when you're out doing your ERP, remind yourself of that very thing. When I am coaching my clients, they often initially feel very anxious about facing the very thing they avoided for so long. However, with time they also are amazed that they are able to sit in the anxiety long enough to realize otherwise.

What is a roadmap?

Here is where you are going to apply what you need to know in order to move forward and start working through your OCD. I like to refer to this as our roadmap, which is your list of things that comprises all your anxiety-provoking items. It might be items such as situations that you fear and avoid; it might be items that are in your thought process; it might be certain objects that are specific events; it may be anything that causes you to have obsessions and therefore have some form of compulsion to alleviate the anxiety.

A roadmap defines the starting and ending points and everything in-between. As your coach, I help you make a list of all the obsessions and compulsions, rating each one with an anxiety rating on a scale of 0-10 or 0-100 with the lowest numbers reflecting low anxiety and higher numbers indicating higher levels of anxiety. It is important to keep in mind the anxiety rating is based on if you were NOT able to perform the compulsion related to that specific obsession. This becomes our foundation and like anything if you want to have a positive outcome and solid structure you first must start with a solid foundation, which is your inventory for ALL of your OCD antagonists.

Courage

Developing a roadmap will take dedication and courage. It is important to remember the definition of courage. Courage is not the absence of fear or despair but the ability to conquer them. Courage is a willingness to take necessary action in the face of fear. Look at your exposure exercises for OCD, as exercises in courage. A long time ago I heard a saying that fear is a story you tell yourself may happen.

The acronym I learned for fear is False Evidence Appearing Real. The more you confront your fear, the more it will dissipate into the air. Let it go.

If you are like me, who spent years responding to the voice of OCD by giving in, here's the problem, I realized the more I gave into it the worse it became. As your coach, I'm able to share ways and means to help prevent you from going through the same ordeal. Imagine how you would feel if you could wake up to the freedom of life's choices rather than the slavery of irrational thought processes.
If you no longer had the limits placed on you by your OCD, what would it look like to have the ability to choose freely, your thoughts. We at The OCD Coach can help you rid yourself of the fears that have paralysed you and bound you like a prisoner in your own body.

In my book, The 6 Secrets To The Deliverance From OCD, there is a step-by-step process that can be learned, implemented, and therefore help you achieve success in breaking the chains from OCD. Invest in yourself today by pre-ordering your copy at a discount, for a limited time.

Get your copy here:

https://theocdcoach.com/best-selling-books

"I'll Meet You There"

Sandra Wallace

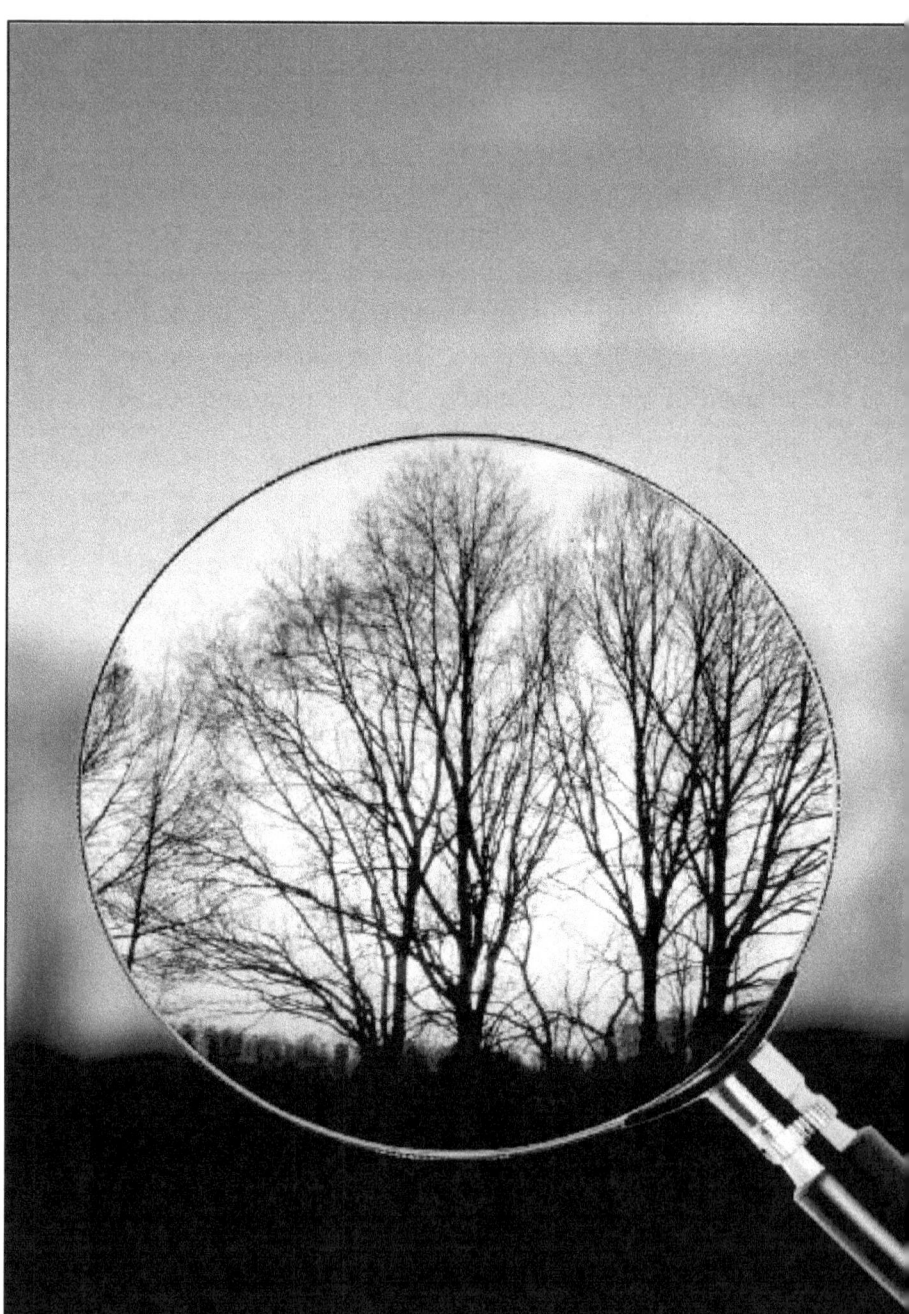

"Having this step-by-step approach helps to identify the signs and symptoms of OCD and therefore allows one to start challenging, facing and overcoming their obsessions and compulsions. Would recommend!"

- Lauren Roskilly, BA, (Hons) Bestselling Author, Mindful of Christ Ministries

"Sandra is so encouraging and inspiring to help others build a better life."

-Dr. Irene Ching, Medical Practitioner

"Sandra provides a simple and proven system to change your thinking and inspire belief in oneself."

- Valerie Heaman, Teacher/Educator

"Sandra is an expert Coach in OCD who has experience in teaching not only coming from the role of a psychiatric nurse but from "obsessing" and "overcoming" the challenges faced in living with her own obsessive-compulsive disorder. Definitely educational for those of us who do not fully understand. In the hopes of supporting anyone who has OCD it's the perfect gift."

- Edith Gagne, Chopra Center Certified Instructor

www.ingramcontent.com/pod-product-compliance
Lightning Source LLC
Chambersburg PA
CBHW070521220526
45467CB00002B/781